# THE LEAKY GUT COOKBOOK

## JULIET HENRY

# INTRODUCTION

Welcome to the world of healing and nourishment! In this book, "The Leaky Gut Cookbook," we embark on a journey of culinary exploration and nutritional empowerment to address one of the most pervasive yet often misunderstood health challenges of our time: leaky gut syndrome.

Leaky gut syndrome, also known as intestinal permeability, is a condition that has garnered increasing attention in recent years within the realm of holistic health and functional medicine. It is a complex and multifaceted disorder characterized by the compromise of the intestinal barrier, leading to the leakage of toxins, undigested food particles, and harmful microbes from the gut into the bloodstream. This breach of the gut barrier triggers an inflammatory response in the body, contributing to a wide array of health issues ranging from digestive discomfort and food sensitivities to autoimmune disorders and chronic inflammation.

While leaky gut syndrome may manifest differently from person to person, its underlying mechanisms underscore the fundamental importance of gut health in maintaining overall well-being. Indeed, the health of our gut microbiome—the vast ecosystem of microorganisms residing within our intestines—plays a pivotal role not only in digestion and nutrient absorption but also in immune function, mood regulation, and even cognitive health.

In the face of modern dietary habits, environmental toxins, chronic stress, and overuse of antibiotics, the prevalence of leaky gut syndrome has soared, affecting millions of individuals worldwide. Yet, amidst the complexity of this condition, there lies a beacon of hope: the transformative power of food as medicine.

"The Leaky Gut Cookbook" is more than just a collection of recipes—it is a testament to the profound impact that mindful, nourishing cuisine can have on our health and vitality. Within these pages, you will discover a treasure trove of delicious, gut-nourishing recipes meticulously crafted to support digestive wellness, reduce inflammation, and restore balance to the body.

From vibrant salads bursting with phytonutrients to comforting soups brimming with healing herbs and spices, each recipe in this cookbook is thoughtfully designed to promote gut healing and enhance overall vitality. Drawing inspiration from diverse culinary traditions and the latest scientific research on gut health, these recipes celebrate the abundance of whole, nutrient-dense foods that nature has to offer.

But "The Leaky Gut Cookbook" is more than just a culinary guide—it is a comprehensive resource that empowers you to reclaim your health and vitality from the inside out. In addition to mouthwatering recipes, you will find practical tips for supporting digestive health, guidance on identifying and avoiding potential trigger foods, and insights into the latest advancements in gut-healing protocols.

Whether you are embarking on your journey to wellness or seeking to deepen your understanding of the intricate interplay between diet and gut health, "The Leaky Gut Cookbook" is your trusted companion on the path to vibrant health and vitality. Let these pages be your roadmap to digestive wellness, as you savor the nourishing flavors of healing cuisine and embrace the transformative power of food as medicine.

So, dear reader, I invite you to embark on this culinary adventure with an open heart and a curious palate. May each recipe you prepare and every meal you enjoy be a celebration of health, healing, and the infinite potential that resides within you. Together, let us nourish our bodies, uplift our spirits, and cultivate a deep and abiding reverence for the miraculous journey of healing that unfolds with every bite.

# CHAPTER ONE

"Leaky gut" refers to a condition characterized by increased permeability of the intestinal lining, allowing substances such as toxins, bacteria, undigested food particles, and other harmful microbes to leak through the lining and enter the bloodstream. In a healthy gut, the lining of the intestines acts as a barrier, selectively allowing nutrients to pass through while keeping harmful substances out. However, when the intestinal lining becomes compromised or "leaky," it can lead to various health issues and inflammatory responses throughout the body.

The intestinal lining is made up of epithelial cells held together by tight junctions. These tight junctions control the permeability of the intestinal barrier, regulating the passage of molecules and substances. When these tight junctions become damaged or weakened, the barrier function is compromised, leading to increased permeability and the leakage of unwanted substances into the bloodstream.

## Factors Can Contribute To The Development Of Leaky Gut Syndrome,

1. **Diet:** A diet high in processed foods, refined sugars, gluten, and other inflammatory foods can contribute to inflammation in the gut and compromise the integrity of the intestinal lining.

2. **Chronic Stress:** Prolonged stress can impair digestive function and weaken the immune system, making the gut more susceptible to inflammation and damage.

3. **Medications**: Certain medications, such as nonsteroidal anti-inflammatory drugs

(NSAIDs), antibiotics, and proton pump inhibitors (PPIs), can disrupt the balance of gut bacteria and contribute to leaky gut syndrome.

4. **Environmental Factors:** Environmental toxins, such as pesticides, heavy metals, and pollutants, can also damage the intestinal lining and contribute to leaky gut.

5. **Imbalance of Gut Microbiota**: An imbalance in the gut microbiota, known as dysbiosis, can disrupt the delicate ecosystem of beneficial bacteria in the gut and contribute to inflammation and leaky gut syndrome.

The consequences of leaky gut syndrome can extend beyond the digestive system and impact various aspects of health, including:

1. **Immune System Dysfunction:** The leakage of toxins and harmful substances into the bloodstream can trigger an immune response, leading to chronic inflammation and autoimmune reactions.

2. **Nutrient Malabsorption:** A compromised intestinal barrier can impair the absorption of essential nutrients, vitamins, and minerals, leading to nutritional deficiencies and related health issues.

3. **Food Sensitivities and Allergies:** Leaky gut syndrome is associated with the development of food sensitivities and allergies, as undigested food particles and antigens leak into the bloodstream and trigger immune reactions.

4. **Chronic Inflammatory Conditions:**
Leaky gut syndrome has been linked to various chronic inflammatory conditions, including irritable bowel syndrome (IBS), inflammatory bowel disease (IBD), rheumatoid arthritis, and autoimmune diseases.

5. **Brain Health:** There is growing evidence to suggest that leaky gut syndrome may play a role in the development of neurological disorders, such as depression, anxiety, and cognitive decline, through the gut-brain axis.

**Leaky Gut Syndrome**

The management of leaky gut syndrome typically involves addressing underlying factors contributing to intestinal permeability, such as dietary changes, stress management, supplementation with probiotics and digestive enzymes, and lifestyle modifications. A leaky gut diet, such as the one outlined in your "Leaky Guts Cookbook," may emphasize nutrient-dense whole foods, gut-healing foods like bone broth, fermented foods, and foods rich in fiber and antioxidants to support gut health and repair the intestinal lining. Additionally, identifying and eliminating potential food triggers and inflammatory substances from the diet can help reduce inflammation and promote healing in the gut. However, it's essential to consult with a healthcare professional or registered dietitian for personalized recommendations and guidance on managing leaky gut syndrome.

Leaky gut syndrome, also known as increased intestinal permeability, is a condition that affects the lining of the intestines. In a healthy intestine, the lining acts as a barrier, allowing nutrients to pass through while preventing harmful substances such as bacteria, toxins, and undigested food particles from entering the bloodstream. However, in individuals with leaky gut syndrome, this barrier becomes compromised, allowing these harmful substances to leak into the bloodstream and trigger an immune response.

The symptoms of leaky gut syndrome can vary widely among individuals and may include:

1. **Digestive issues:** Symptoms such as bloating, gas, diarrhea, constipation, and abdominal pain are common in individuals with leaky gut syndrome. The compromised intestinal lining can disrupt the normal digestive process, leading to these symptoms.

2. **Food sensitivities**: Leaky gut syndrome is associated with the development of food sensitivities and intolerances. When undigested food particles leak into the

bloodstream, the immune system may recognize them as foreign invaders and mount an immune response, leading to food sensitivities and allergic reactions.

3. **Inflammation**: The leakage of harmful substances into the bloodstream can trigger an inflammatory response throughout the body. Chronic inflammation is associated with various health problems, including autoimmune disorders, arthritis, and inflammatory bowel diseases.

4. **Fatigue and low energy:** Chronic inflammation and digestive issues can contribute to fatigue and low energy levels in individuals with leaky gut syndrome. The body may divert energy resources to fight inflammation and repair the intestinal lining, leading to feelings of fatigue and lethargy.

5. **Joint pain and muscle aches:** Inflammatory cytokines released in response to leaky gut syndrome can contribute to joint pain and muscle aches. These symptoms may mimic those of autoimmune disorders such as rheumatoid arthritis.

6. **Skin problems:** Leaky gut syndrome has been linked to skin conditions such as acne, eczema, and psoriasis. The immune system's response to circulating toxins and inflammatory molecules may manifest as skin inflammation and irritation.

7. **Autoimmune disorders: Some researchers** believe that leaky gut syndrome may contribute to the development of autoimmune disorders. When the immune system becomes dysregulated due to chronic inflammation and exposure to harmful

substances, it may mistakenly attack healthy tissues and organs.

The impact of leaky gut syndrome extends beyond physical symptoms and can affect an individual's overall health and well-being. Chronic inflammation and immune dysregulation associated with leaky gut syndrome may increase the risk of developing other serious health conditions, including cardiovascular disease, diabetes, and neurological disorders.

Nutrition plays a pivotal role in managing leaky gut syndrome, and your book, "Leaky Guts Cookbook," could serve as an invaluable resource for individuals seeking to address this condition through dietary means. Leaky gut syndrome, also known as increased intestinal permeability, is a condition characterized by a compromised intestinal barrier that allows toxins, bacteria, and undigested food particles to leak into the bloodstream, triggering inflammation and immune system responses. Nutrition can both exacerbate and ameliorate this condition, making dietary interventions a crucial component of leaky gut management.

## The Role Of Nutrition In Managing Leaky Gut Syndrome:

1. **Identifying Trigger Foods:** Your cookbook can help individuals identify and eliminate foods that contribute to intestinal inflammation and permeability. Common trigger foods include gluten, dairy, processed sugars, artificial additives, and refined carbohydrates. By providing recipes free from these potential irritants, individuals can begin to heal their gut and reduce inflammation.

2. **Promoting Gut Healing Foods:** Incorporating nutrient-dense, whole foods is essential for promoting gut healing. Your cookbook can emphasize foods rich in antioxidants, vitamins, minerals, and phytonutrients, such as fruits, vegetables, lean proteins, healthy fats, and fermented foods. These foods can support the repair of the intestinal lining and enhance overall gut health.

3. **Emphasizing Gut-Supportive Nutrients:** Certain nutrients play key roles in gut health and can be incorporated into recipes featured in your cookbook. For example:

- Omega-3 Fatty Acids: Found in fatty fish, flaxseeds, chia seeds, and walnuts, omega-3 fatty acids possess anti-inflammatory properties that can help reduce intestinal inflammation.

- Glutamine: An amino acid critical for intestinal cell regeneration and repair, glutamine can be sourced from foods like bone broth, spinach, cabbage, and parsley.

- Zinc: Essential for maintaining intestinal barrier function and immune system health, zinc-rich foods such as shellfish, pumpkin seeds, and legumes can be included in recipes.

- Quercetin: A flavonoid with anti-inflammatory properties, quercetin is abundant in foods like apples, onions, berries, and citrus fruits.

4. **Emphasizing Gut-Supportive Supplements:** In addition to dietary interventions, supplements may complement leaky gut management. Your cookbook can provide guidance on incorporating gut-supportive supplements such as probiotics, prebiotics, digestive enzymes, and L-

glutamine into recipes or as adjuncts to meals.

5. **Encouraging Hydration and Fiber Intake:** Adequate hydration and fiber intake are essential for maintaining regular bowel movements and supporting the growth of beneficial gut bacteria. Recipes in your cookbook can include hydrating ingredients like cucumber, watermelon, and herbal teas, as well as fiber-rich foods such as whole grains, legumes, nuts, seeds, and vegetables.

6. **Emphasizing Proper Food Preparation Methods**: Certain cooking methods can enhance nutrient absorption and digestibility while minimizing potential gut irritants. Your cookbook can promote gentle cooking techniques like steaming, roasting, and sautéing, which preserve the nutritional

integrity of ingredients and may be easier on the digestive system.

7. **Addressing Individual Nutrient Needs**: Nutritional requirements vary among individuals, and factors such as age, gender, genetics, and underlying health conditions can influence nutrient needs. Your cookbook can provide general dietary recommendations while encouraging readers to consult with healthcare professionals or registered dietitians to personalize their nutritional approach to managing leaky gut syndrome.

8. **Encouraging Mindful Eating Practices:** Beyond the specific foods and nutrients consumed, your cookbook can promote mindful eating practices such as chewing food thoroughly, eating in a relaxed environment, and paying attention to hunger

and satiety cues. These practices can support optimal digestion and nutrient absorption while reducing the risk of gastrointestinal discomfort.

## Understanding which foods to avoid for individuals with leaky gut syndrome

It is essential for managing symptoms and promoting gut healing. Leaky gut, also known as increased intestinal permeability, is a condition where the lining of the intestines becomes damaged, allowing undigested food particles, toxins, and bacteria to leak into the bloodstream, triggering inflammation and various health issues.

1. **Gluten-containing grains**: Wheat, barley, rye, and products made from them contain gluten, which can be difficult to digest and may contribute to intestinal inflammation.

2. **Dairy products**: Cow's milk and dairy products containing lactose can be problematic for individuals with leaky gut due to lactose intolerance and the potential for dairy proteins to trigger inflammation.

3. **Refined sugars and artificial sweeteners:** Highly processed sugars and artificial sweeteners can disrupt gut flora balance and contribute to inflammation. Avoid foods high in sucrose, fructose, and corn syrup.

4. **Processed foods:** Processed foods often contain artificial additives, preservatives,

and unhealthy fats that can irritate the gut lining and promote inflammation. This includes packaged snacks, fast food, and pre-packaged meals.

5. **Highly processed oils:** Vegetable oils like soybean oil, corn oil, and sunflower oil are often high in omega-6 fatty acids, which can promote inflammation when consumed in excess. Opt for healthier fats like olive oil, avocado oil, and coconut oil instead.

6. **Alcohol:** Alcohol can disrupt the balance of gut bacteria and increase intestinal permeability, leading to inflammation and aggravating leaky gut symptoms. It's best to avoid or limit alcohol consumption.

7. Caffeine: Caffeine can stimulate the production of stomach acid and may irritate

the gastrointestinal tract in some individuals. Limiting or avoiding caffeinated beverages like coffee, tea, and energy drinks may be beneficial.

8. **Spicy foods:** Spicy foods can irritate the gastrointestinal tract and exacerbate symptoms such as heartburn and acid reflux. Avoiding foods high in spices and capsaicin can help reduce discomfort.

9. **Nightshade vegetables**: Some individuals with leaky gut syndrome may be sensitive to nightshade vegetables like tomatoes, peppers, eggplants, and potatoes, which contain compounds known as alkaloids that may contribute to inflammation in sensitive individuals.

10. **Highly acidic foods:** Foods that are highly acidic, such as citrus fruits and vinegar, can aggravate gastrointestinal symptoms in some individuals. It may be helpful to reduce consumption of acidic foods and beverages.

11. **Artificial additives and preservatives:** Foods containing artificial additives, preservatives, and food colorings can disrupt gut health and contribute to inflammation. Reading food labels and choosing whole, minimally processed foods is recommended.

12. **Allergenic foods:** Individuals with leaky gut may have sensitivities or allergies to certain foods such as nuts, shellfish, and eggs. Identifying and avoiding allergenic foods can help reduce inflammation and improve symptoms.

By focusing on whole, nutrient-dense foods and avoiding processed, inflammatory foods, individuals with leaky gut syndrome can support gut healing and improve overall health. "Leaky Guts Cookbook" can provide delicious and nourishing recipes that adhere to these dietary principles, helping readers manage their symptoms and promote gut health.

# CHAPTER TWO

## LEAKY GUT RECIPES

### 1. Gut-Healing Smoothie Bowl:

Ingredients:

- 1 cup mixed berries (blueberries, strawberries, raspberries)

- 1 banana

- 1 cup almond milk

- 1 tablespoon chia seeds

- 1 tablespoon flaxseeds

- 1 tablespoon hemp seeds

- 1/2 cup Greek yogurt (optional)

Instructions:

1. Blend all ingredients until smooth.

2. Pour into a bowl and top with additional berries, nuts, and seeds.

## 2. Quinoa and Vegetable Stuffed Peppers:

Ingredients:

- 4 bell peppers, halved

- 1 cup cooked quinoa

- 1 cup black beans, rinsed and drained

- 1 cup diced tomatoes

- 1 cup chopped spinach

- 1 teaspoon cumin

- 1 teaspoon paprika

- Salt and pepper to taste

Instructions:

1. Preheat oven to 375°F (190°C).

2. Mix all ingredients in a bowl.

3. Stuff the pepper halves with the mixture.

4. Bake for 25-30 minutes until peppers are tender.

## 3. Turmeric and Ginger Carrot Soup:

Ingredients:

- 1 pound carrots, chopped

- 1 onion, diced

- 2 cloves garlic, minced

- 1 tablespoon fresh ginger, grated

- 1 teaspoon turmeric powder

- 4 cups vegetable broth

- Salt and pepper to taste

- 1 tablespoon coconut oil

Instructions:

1. In a pot, sauté onions, garlic, and ginger in coconut oil until softened.

2. Add carrots, turmeric, and vegetable broth. Bring to a boil.

3. Simmer until carrots are tender.

4. Blend until smooth. Season with salt and pepper.

## 4. Salmon and Avocado Nori Wraps:

Ingredients:

- 4 sheets nori seaweed

- 8 ounces cooked salmon, flaked

- 1 avocado, sliced

- 1 cucumber, julienned

- 1 tablespoon tamari sauce

- Sesame seeds for garnish

Instructions:

1. Place a nori sheet on a bamboo sushi rolling mat.

2. Spread salmon, avocado, and cucumber evenly.

3. Roll tightly and seal the edge with tamari sauce.

4. Slice into bite-sized pieces. Sprinkle with sesame seeds.

## 5. Chickpea and Spinach Coconut Curry:

Ingredients:

- 1 can chickpeas, drained and rinsed

- 2 cups spinach, chopped

- 1 can coconut milk

- 1 onion, diced

- 2 cloves garlic, minced

- 1 tablespoon curry powder

- 1 teaspoon turmeric powder

- Salt and pepper to taste

Instructions:

1. Sauté onions and garlic in a pot until translucent.

2. Add chickpeas, spinach, coconut milk, and spices.

3. Simmer until spinach wilts. Season with salt and pepper.

## 6. Gut-Healing Bone Broth:

Ingredients:

- 2-3 pounds beef bones (grass-fed, organic)

- 1 onion, quartered

- 2 carrots, chopped

- 2 celery stalks, chopped

- 4 cloves garlic, smashed

- 2 tablespoons apple cider vinegar

- Water to cover bones

- Salt and pepper to taste

Instructions:

1. Place bones, vegetables, and apple cider vinegar in a large pot.

2. Cover with water and bring to a boil. Skim off any foam.

3. Reduce heat to low and simmer for 12-24 hours.

4. Strain broth and season with salt and pepper.

## 7. Zucchini Noodles with Pesto:

Ingredients:

- 4 medium zucchinis, spiralized

- 1 cup fresh basil leaves

- 1/4 cup pine nuts

- 2 cloves garlic

- 1/4 cup olive oil

- Juice of 1 lemon

- Salt and pepper to taste

- Optional: grated Parmesan cheese

Instructions:

1. In a food processor, blend basil, pine nuts, garlic, olive oil, and lemon juice until smooth.

2. Season with salt and pepper.

3. Toss zucchini noodles with pesto until well coated.

4. Serve with grated Parmesan cheese if desired.

## 8. Gut-Healing Chicken and Vegetable Stir-Fry:

Ingredients:

- 1 lb chicken breast, thinly sliced

- 2 cups mixed vegetables (bell peppers, broccoli, snap peas)

- 2 cloves garlic, minced

- 1 tablespoon ginger, minced

- 2 tablespoons coconut aminos

- 1 tablespoon sesame oil

- 2 tablespoons avocado oil

- Salt and pepper to taste


Instructions:

1. Heat avocado oil in a large skillet over medium-high heat.

2. Add chicken and cook until browned and cooked through.

3. Add garlic and ginger, cook for 1 minute.

4. Add mixed vegetables and cook until tender-crisp.

5. Stir in coconut aminos and sesame oil. Season with salt and pepper.

# 9. Gut-Healing Chia Seed Pudding:

Ingredients:

- 1/4 cup chia seeds

- 1 cup almond milk

- 1 teaspoon vanilla extract

- 1 tablespoon honey or maple syrup (optional)

- Fresh berries for topping

Instructions:

1. In a bowl, mix chia seeds, almond milk, vanilla extract, and sweetener (if using).

2. Stir well and let sit for 5 minutes. Stir again to prevent clumping.

3. Cover and refrigerate for at least 2 hours or overnight.

4. Serve topped with fresh berries.

## 10. Roasted Root Vegetables:

Ingredients:

- 2 carrots, peeled and diced

- 2 parsnips, peeled and diced

- 2 sweet potatoes, peeled and diced

- 2 tablespoons olive oil

- 1 teaspoon dried thyme

- Salt and pepper to taste

Instructions:

1. Preheat oven to 400°F (200°C).

2. Toss diced vegetables with olive oil, thyme, salt, and pepper.

3. Spread vegetables in a single layer on a baking sheet.

4. Roast for 25-30 minutes until vegetables are tender and caramelized.

## 11. Gut-Healing Turkey and Vegetable Soup:

Ingredients:

- 1 lb ground turkey

- 4 cups chicken or vegetable broth

- 2 carrots, diced

- 2 celery stalks, diced

- 1 onion, diced

- 2 cloves garlic, minced

- 1 teaspoon dried thyme

- Salt and pepper to taste

- Fresh parsley for garnish

Instructions:

1. In a large pot, brown ground turkey over medium heat.

2. Add onions, garlic, carrots, and celery. Cook until vegetables are tender.

3. Pour in chicken or vegetable broth and add thyme, salt, and pepper.

4. Simmer for 20-25 minutes.

5. Garnish with fresh parsley before serving.

## 12. Gut-Healing Coconut Flour Pancakes:

Ingredients:

- 1/4 cup coconut flour

- 4 eggs

- 1/4 cup coconut milk

- 1 tablespoon honey or maple syrup (optional)

- 1/2 teaspoon baking powder

- Pinch of salt

- Coconut oil for cooking

Instructions:

1. In a bowl, whisk together eggs, coconut milk, and honey/maple syrup.

2. Add coconut flour, baking powder, and salt. Mix until well combined.

3. Heat coconut oil in a skillet over medium heat.

4. Pour batter onto the skillet to form pancakes.

5. Cook until bubbles form on the surface, then flip and cook until golden brown.

6. Serve with fresh fruit or pure maple syrup.

## 13. Gut-Healing Cucumber Avocado Salad:

Ingredients:

- 2 cucumbers, thinly sliced

- 1 avocado, diced

- 1/4 cup red onion, thinly sliced

- 2 tablespoons fresh cilantro, chopped

- Juice of 1 lime

- 1 tablespoon olive oil

- Salt and pepper to taste

Instructions:

1. In a large bowl, combine cucumbers, avocado, red onion, and cilantro.

2. Drizzle with lime juice and olive oil.

3. Season with salt and pepper. Toss gently to combine.

4. Serve chilled.

## 14. Gut-Healing Baked Salmon with Lemon and Dill:

Ingredients:

- 4 salmon fillets

- 2 tablespoons olive oil

- 2 tablespoons fresh dill, chopped

- 2 cloves garlic, minced

- Juice of 1 lemon

- Salt and pepper to taste

Instructions:

1. Preheat oven to 375°F (190°C).

2. Place salmon fillets on a baking sheet lined with parchment paper.

3. In a small bowl, mix olive oil, dill, garlic, lemon juice, salt, and pepper.

4. Brush the mixture over the salmon fillets.

5. Bake for 12-15 minutes or until salmon is cooked through and flakes easily with a fork.

6. Serve with additional lemon wedges if desired.

## 15. Gut-Healing Green Detox Smoothie:

Ingredients:

- 1 cup spinach

- 1/2 cup kale

- 1/2 cucumber, chopped

- 1 green apple, cored and chopped

- 1/2 lemon, juiced

- 1-inch piece of ginger, peeled

- 1 cup coconut water or almond milk

- Ice cubes (optional)


Instructions:

1. Blend all ingredients until smooth.

2. Add ice cubes if desired for a colder smoothie.

3. Serve immediately.

## 16. Gut-Healing Miso Soup:

Ingredients:

- 4 cups water or vegetable broth

- 2 tablespoons miso paste

- 1 block tofu, diced

- 2 green onions, thinly sliced

- 1 sheet nori, cut into thin strips

- 1 tablespoon soy sauce or tamari

- 1 teaspoon sesame oil

- Optional: sliced mushrooms, spinach, or wakame seaweed

Instructions:

1. In a pot, bring water or vegetable broth to a simmer.

2. Dissolve miso paste in a small bowl with some warm water from the pot.

3. Add tofu, green onions, nori, soy sauce, and any optional ingredients to the pot.

4. Simmer for 5-10 minutes.

5. Stir in sesame oil before serving.


## 17. Gut-Healing Almond Flour Banana Bread:

Ingredients:

- 2 ripe bananas, mashed

- 3 eggs

- 1/4 cup coconut oil, melted

- 1/4 cup honey or maple syrup

- 1 teaspoon vanilla extract

- 2 cups almond flour

- 1 teaspoon baking powder

- 1/2 teaspoon cinnamon

- Pinch of salt

- Optional: chopped nuts or dark chocolate chips

Instructions:

1. Preheat oven to 350°F (175°C). Grease a loaf pan with coconut oil.

2. In a bowl, mix mashed bananas, eggs, coconut oil, honey/maple syrup, and vanilla extract.

3. Add almond flour, baking powder, cinnamon, and salt. Mix until well combined.

4. Fold in chopped nuts or dark chocolate chips if using.

5. Pour batter into the prepared loaf pan.

6. Bake for 45-50 minutes or until a toothpick inserted into the center comes out clean.

7. Let cool before slicing.

## 18. Gut-Healing Lentil Salad:

Ingredients:

- 1 cup cooked lentils

- 1 cucumber, diced

- 1 bell pepper, diced

- 1/4 red onion, finely chopped

- 1/4 cup fresh parsley, chopped

- Juice of 1 lemon

- 2 tablespoons olive oil

- Salt and pepper to taste

Instructions:

1. In a large bowl, combine cooked lentils, cucumber, bell pepper, red onion, and parsley.

2. Drizzle lemon juice and olive oil over the salad.

3. Season with salt and pepper. Toss gently to combine.

4. Serve chilled or at room temperature.

## 19. Gut-Healing Sweet Potato and Kale Hash:

Ingredients:

- 2 sweet potatoes, peeled and diced

- 2 cups kale, chopped

- 1 onion, diced

- 2 cloves garlic, minced

- 2 tablespoons olive oil

- 1 teaspoon paprika

- Salt and pepper to taste

Instructions:

1. Heat olive oil in a skillet over medium heat.

2. Add diced sweet potatoes and cook until tender, about 10 minutes.

3. Add onions and garlic, cook until softened.

4. Stir in chopped kale and paprika. Cook until kale is wilted.

5. Season with salt and pepper before serving.

## 20. Gut-Healing Roasted Brussels Sprouts:

Ingredients:

- 1 lb Brussels sprouts, trimmed and halved

- 2 tablespoons olive oil

- 2 cloves garlic, minced

- 1 teaspoon lemon zest

- Salt and pepper to taste

Instructions:

1. Preheat oven to 400°F (200°C).

2. Toss Brussels sprouts with olive oil, garlic, lemon zest, salt, and pepper.

3. Spread Brussels sprouts in a single layer on a baking sheet.

4. Roast for 20-25 minutes until browned and crispy.

5. Serve hot.

These recipes offer nutritious options to support gut health and provide a variety of flavors to enjoy. Let me know if you'd like more recipes or have any other questions!

## 21. Gut-Healing Chicken and Vegetable Kebabs:

Ingredients:

- 1 lb chicken breast, cut into chunks

- 2 bell peppers, cut into chunks

- 1 red onion, cut into chunks

- 8 cherry tomatoes

- 2 tablespoons olive oil

- 2 cloves garlic, minced

- 1 teaspoon paprika

- 1 teaspoon cumin

- Salt and pepper to taste

- Wooden skewers, soaked in water


Instructions:

1. In a bowl, mix olive oil, minced garlic, paprika, cumin, salt, and pepper.

2. Thread chicken, bell peppers, red onion, and cherry tomatoes onto skewers.

3. Brush the skewers with the olive oil mixture.

4. Grill kebabs over medium heat for 10-12 minutes, turning occasionally, until chicken is cooked through and vegetables are tender.

## 22. Gut-Healing Cauliflower Rice Stir-Fry:

Ingredients:

- 1 head cauliflower, grated into rice-like texture

- 2 carrots, diced

- 1 bell pepper, diced

- 1 cup snap peas

- 2 cloves garlic, minced

- 2 tablespoons coconut aminos or soy sauce

- 1 tablespoon sesame oil

- 2 green onions, thinly sliced

- Salt and pepper to taste

Instructions:

1. In a large skillet or wok, heat sesame oil over medium heat.

2. Add minced garlic and cook until fragrant.

3. Add diced carrots, bell pepper, and snap peas. Stir-fry for 3-4 minutes until vegetables are tender-crisp.

4. Add cauliflower rice and coconut aminos or soy sauce. Cook for another 3-4 minutes, stirring constantly.

5. Season with salt and pepper. Garnish with sliced green onions before serving.

# 23. Gut-Healing Blueberry Oatmeal Breakfast Bowl:

Ingredients:

- 1/2 cup rolled oats

- 1 cup almond milk

- 1/2 teaspoon cinnamon

- 1/2 cup fresh blueberries

- 1 tablespoon almond butter

- 1 tablespoon honey or maple syrup (optional)

- Sliced almonds for garnish


Instructions:

1. In a saucepan, combine rolled oats, almond milk, and cinnamon.

2. Cook over medium heat, stirring occasionally, until oats are tender and creamy.

3. Stir in fresh blueberries and almond butter.

4. Sweeten with honey or maple syrup if desired.

5. Serve hot, garnished with sliced almonds.

## 24. Gut-Healing Spinach and Feta Stuffed Chicken Breast:

Ingredients:

- 4 boneless, skinless chicken breasts

- 2 cups fresh spinach leaves

- 1/2 cup crumbled feta cheese

- 2 cloves garlic, minced

- 1 tablespoon olive oil

- Salt and pepper to taste

Instructions:

1. Preheat oven to 375°F (190°C).

2. In a skillet, heat olive oil over medium heat. Add minced garlic and cook until fragrant.

3. Add fresh spinach leaves and cook until wilted. Remove from heat and let cool slightly.

4. Stir in crumbled feta cheese. Season with salt and pepper.

5. Cut a pocket into each chicken breast and stuff with the spinach and feta mixture.

6. Secure with toothpicks if necessary.

7. Place stuffed chicken breasts in a baking dish and bake for 25-30 minutes until chicken is cooked through.

## 25. Gut-Healing Coconut Chia Seed Pudding:

Ingredients:

- 1/4 cup chia seeds

- 1 cup coconut milk

- 1 tablespoon honey or maple syrup

- 1/2 teaspoon vanilla extract

- Unsweetened shredded coconut for garnish

- Sliced strawberries for garnish

Instructions:

1. In a bowl, mix chia seeds, coconut milk, honey/maple syrup, and vanilla extract.

2. Stir well and let sit for 5 minutes. Stir again to prevent clumping.

3. Cover and refrigerate for at least 2 hours or overnight.

4. Serve topped with unsweetened shredded coconut and sliced strawberries.

## 26. Gut-Healing Quinoa Salad with Lemon-Herb Dressing:

Ingredients:

- 1 cup quinoa, rinsed

- 2 cups water or vegetable broth

- 1 cucumber, diced

- 1 bell pepper, diced

- 1/4 cup red onion, finely chopped

- 1/4 cup fresh parsley, chopped

- Juice of 2 lemons

- 3 tablespoons olive oil

- 1 tablespoon fresh basil, chopped

- Salt and pepper to taste


Instructions:

1. In a medium saucepan, combine quinoa and water or vegetable broth. Bring to a boil,

then reduce heat and simmer for 15-20 minutes until quinoa is cooked and liquid is absorbed.

2. In a large bowl, combine cooked quinoa, diced cucumber, bell pepper, red onion, and fresh parsley.

3. In a small bowl, whisk together lemon juice, olive oil, fresh basil, salt, and pepper to make the dressing.

4. Pour the dressing over the quinoa salad and toss to coat evenly.

5. Serve chilled or at room temperature.

## 27. Gut-Healing Turkey and Kale Meatballs:

Ingredients:

- 1 lb ground turkey

- 2 cups chopped kale leaves

- 1/4 cup almond flour

- 1 egg

- 2 cloves garlic, minced

- 1 teaspoon dried oregano

- 1 teaspoon dried thyme

- Salt and pepper to taste

- Olive oil for cooking


Instructions:

1. Preheat oven to 375°F (190°C). Line a baking sheet with parchment paper.

2. In a large bowl, combine ground turkey, chopped kale, almond flour, egg, minced garlic, dried oregano, dried thyme, salt, and pepper.

3. Mix until well combined, then form the mixture into meatballs.

4. Place the meatballs on the prepared baking sheet.

5. Bake for 20-25 minutes until meatballs are cooked through and browned.

6. Serve with your favorite sauce or dip.

## 28. Gut-Healing Roasted Garlic Cauliflower Mash:

Ingredients:

- 1 head cauliflower, chopped into florets

- 4 cloves garlic, peeled

- 2 tablespoons olive oil

- Salt and pepper to taste

- Fresh parsley for garnish (optional)

Instructions:

1. Preheat oven to 400°F (200°C). Line a baking sheet with parchment paper.

2. In a large bowl, toss cauliflower florets and garlic cloves with olive oil, salt, and pepper until evenly coated.

3. Spread the cauliflower and garlic on the prepared baking sheet.

4. Roast for 25-30 minutes until cauliflower is tender and lightly browned.

5. Transfer the roasted cauliflower and garlic to a food processor and blend until smooth.

6. Season with additional salt and pepper if needed.

7. Garnish with fresh parsley before serving.

## 29. Gut-Healing Cabbage and Apple Slaw:

Ingredients:

- 4 cups shredded cabbage

- 1 apple, thinly sliced

- 1/4 cup sliced almonds

- 2 tablespoons apple cider vinegar

- 1 tablespoon olive oil

- 1 teaspoon honey

- Salt and pepper to taste

Instructions:

1. In a large bowl, combine shredded cabbage, sliced apple, and sliced almonds.

2. In a small bowl, whisk together apple cider vinegar, olive oil, honey, salt, and pepper to make the dressing.

3. Pour the dressing over the cabbage and apple mixture. Toss until evenly coated.

4. Serve chilled as a refreshing side dish.

## 30. Gut-Healing Baked Cod with Lemon and Herbs:

Ingredients:

- 4 cod fillets

- 2 tablespoons olive oil

- 2 cloves garlic, minced

- Zest of 1 lemon

- 1 tablespoon fresh parsley, chopped

- 1 tablespoon fresh dill, chopped

- Salt and pepper to taste

- Lemon wedges for serving

Instructions:

1. Preheat oven to 375°F (190°C). Line a baking dish with parchment paper.

2. Place cod fillets in the prepared baking dish.

3. In a small bowl, whisk together olive oil, minced garlic, lemon zest, chopped parsley, chopped dill, salt, and pepper.

4. Spoon the herb mixture over the cod fillets, spreading evenly.

5. Bake for 15-20 minutes until fish is opaque and flakes easily with a fork.

6. Serve with lemon wedges for squeezing over the fish.

## 31. Gut-Healing Vegetable and Lentil Soup:

Ingredients:

- 1 cup green or brown lentils, rinsed

- 4 cups vegetable broth

- 1 onion, diced

- 2 carrots, diced

- 2 celery stalks, diced

- 2 cloves garlic, minced

- 1 teaspoon cumin

- 1 teaspoon turmeric

- Salt and pepper to taste

- Fresh parsley for garnish

Instructions:

1. In a large pot, combine lentils, vegetable broth, onion, carrots, celery, garlic, cumin, turmeric, salt, and pepper.

2. Bring the mixture to a boil, then reduce heat to low and simmer for about 25-30 minutes, or until the lentils and vegetables are tender.

3. Adjust seasoning with additional salt and pepper if needed.

4. Serve hot, garnished with fresh parsley.

## 32. Gut-Healing Mediterranean Quinoa Salad:

Ingredients:

- 1 cup cooked quinoa

- 1 cucumber, diced

- 1 bell pepper, diced

- 1/4 cup Kalamata olives, sliced

- 1/4 cup crumbled feta cheese

- 2 tablespoons fresh lemon juice

- 2 tablespoons extra virgin olive oil

- 1 tablespoon fresh parsley, chopped

- Salt and pepper to taste

Instructions:

1. In a large bowl, combine cooked quinoa, diced cucumber, diced bell pepper, sliced Kalamata olives, and crumbled feta cheese.

2. In a small bowl, whisk together lemon juice, olive oil, chopped parsley, salt, and pepper to make the dressing.

3. Pour the dressing over the quinoa salad and toss to combine.

4. Serve chilled or at room temperature.

## 33. Gut-Healing Stir-Fried Bok Choy:

Ingredients:

- 4 baby bok choy, halved lengthwise

- 2 tablespoons coconut oil

- 2 cloves garlic, minced

- 1 teaspoon grated ginger

- 1 tablespoon soy sauce or tamari

- 1 teaspoon sesame oil

- Sesame seeds for garnish

Instructions:

1. Heat coconut oil in a large skillet or wok over medium heat.

2. Add minced garlic and grated ginger, and sauté for 1 minute until fragrant.

3. Add halved baby bok choy to the skillet and stir-fry for 3-4 minutes until tender-crisp.

4. Drizzle soy sauce or tamari and sesame oil over the bok choy, and toss to coat evenly.

5. Remove from heat and transfer to a serving dish.

6. Garnish with sesame seeds before serving.

## 34. Gut-Healing Turmeric Ginger Tea:

Ingredients:

- 1-inch piece of fresh ginger, sliced

- 1 teaspoon ground turmeric

- 4 cups water

- Honey or maple syrup to taste

- Lemon slices for garnish (optional)


Instructions:

1. In a pot, combine sliced ginger, ground turmeric, and water.

2. Bring the mixture to a boil, then reduce heat and simmer for 10-15 minutes.

3. Strain the tea into mugs and sweeten with honey or maple syrup to taste.

4. Garnish with lemon slices if desired.

5. Serve hot and enjoy the soothing benefits of turmeric ginger tea.

## 35. Gut-Healing Stuffed Bell Peppers:

Ingredients:

- 4 bell peppers, halved and seeds removed

- 1 cup cooked quinoa

- 1 can black beans, rinsed and drained

- 1 cup diced tomatoes

- 1 cup chopped spinach

- 1 teaspoon cumin

- 1 teaspoon paprika

- Salt and pepper to taste

- Shredded cheese for topping (optional)

Instructions:

1. Preheat oven to 375°F (190°C).

2. In a large bowl, mix cooked quinoa, black beans, diced tomatoes, chopped spinach, cumin, paprika, salt, and pepper.

3. Spoon the quinoa mixture into each halved bell pepper.

4. Place the stuffed bell peppers in a baking dish.

5. Cover with foil and bake for 25-30 minutes.

6. If desired, remove foil, sprinkle shredded cheese on top of each stuffed pepper, and bake for an additional 5 minutes or until the cheese is melted and bubbly.

7. Serve hot and enjoy the flavorful stuffed bell peppers.

# CONCLUSION

The journey through the "Leaky Gut Cookbook," it's evident that the path to healing begins with the nourishment we provide our bodies. As we've explored the intricate relationship between gut health and overall well-being, we've uncovered a wealth of delicious recipes, insightful tips, and empowering strategies.

From vibrant salads bursting with nutrients to hearty soups brimming with flavor, each dish has been crafted with the intention of nurturing not just our bodies, but our souls. Through the power of wholesome ingredients and mindful cooking, we've discovered that healing is not merely a destination but a continuous, enriching process.

As we bid farewell to these pages, let us carry forth the lessons learned within them. Let us approach each meal with intention, savoring the goodness it offers us both physically and spiritually. Let us remember that in nourishing our bodies, we nurture our vitality, our resilience, and our capacity for joy.

May this cookbook serve as a guiding light on your journey to optimal health and vitality. May you continue to explore, to experiment, and to savor the abundance that life has to offer. And may you always remember that true wellness begins from within, one delicious bite at a time.